ANATOMY Coloring Book

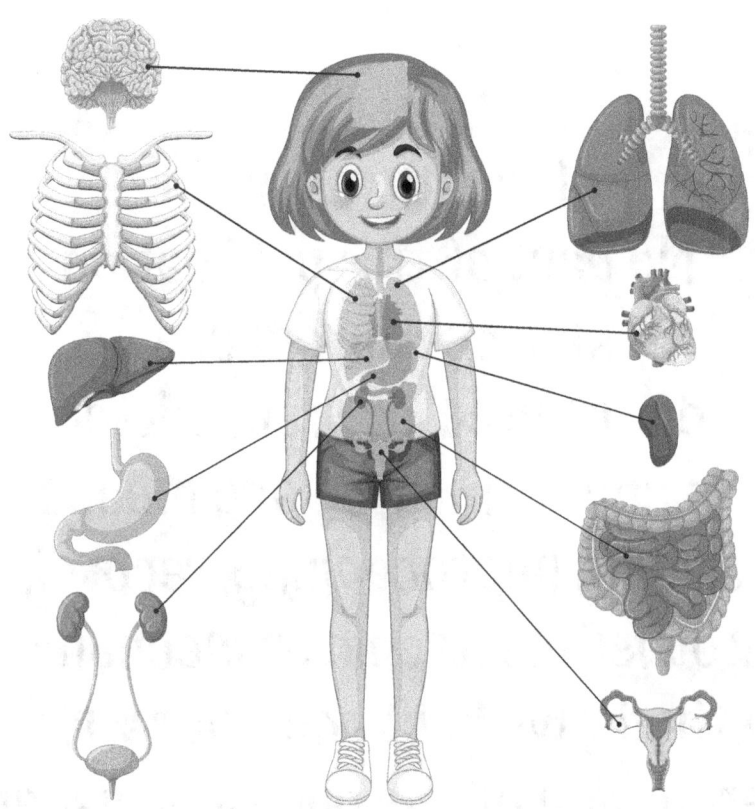

This Book Belongs To

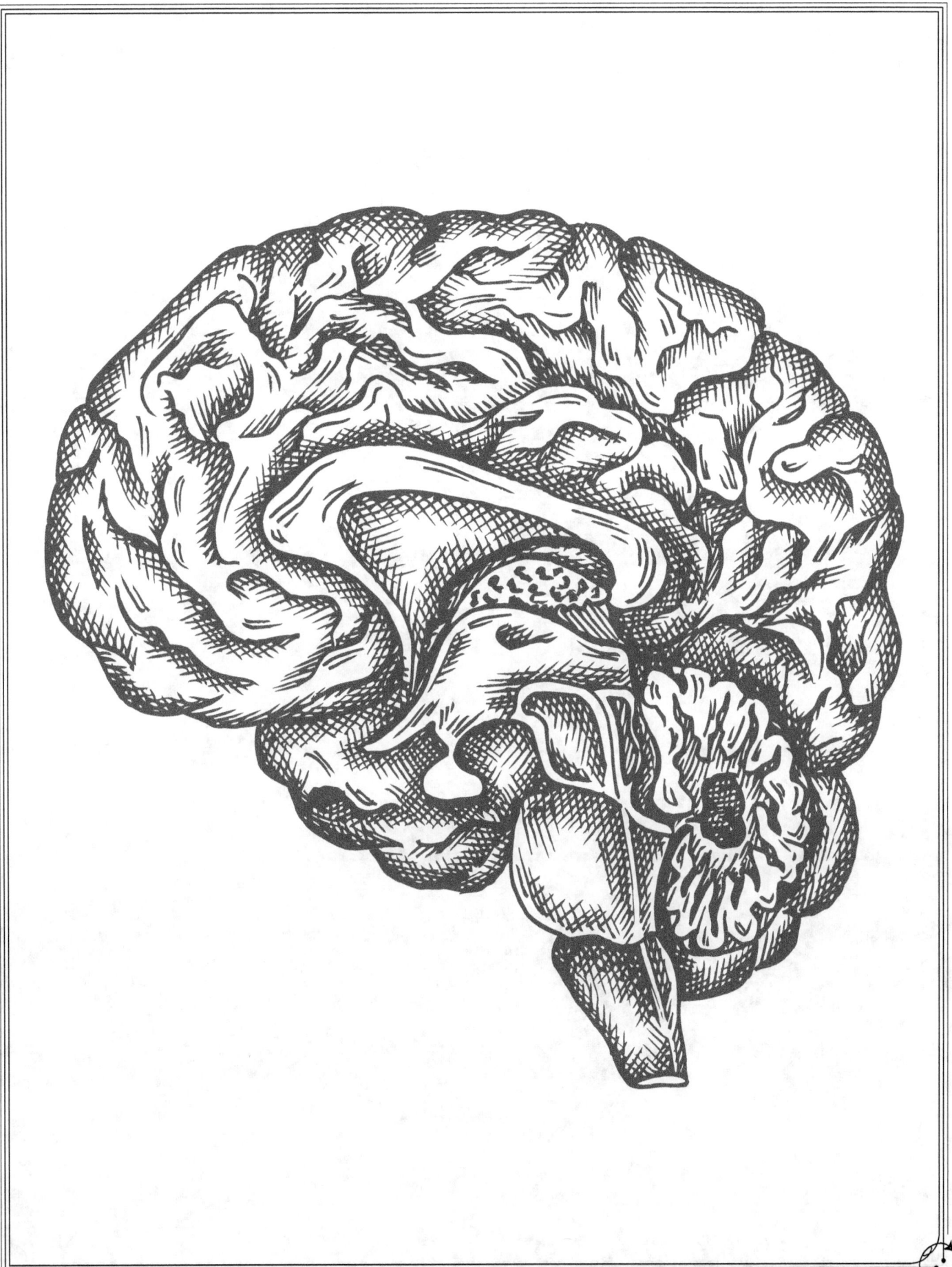

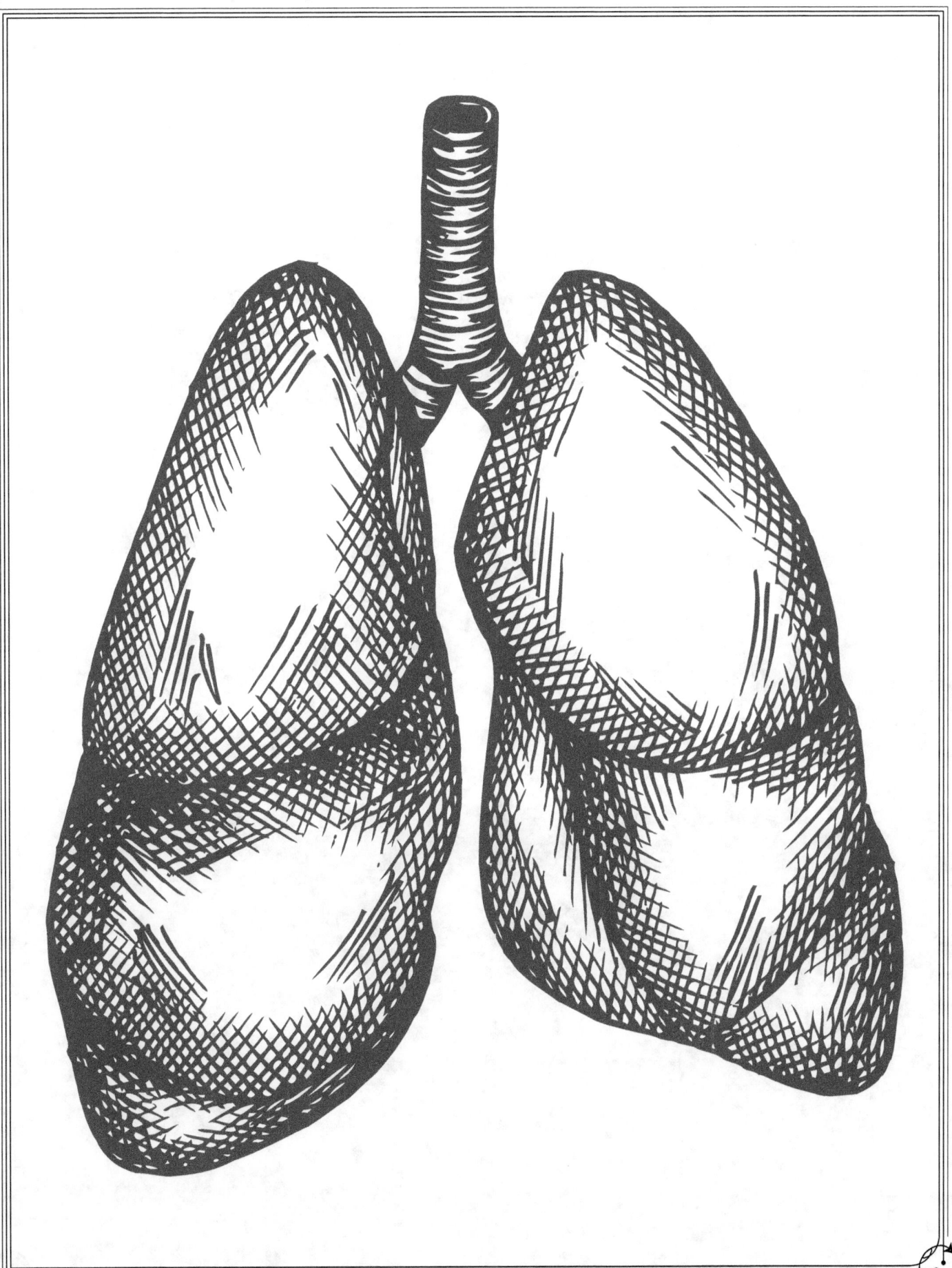

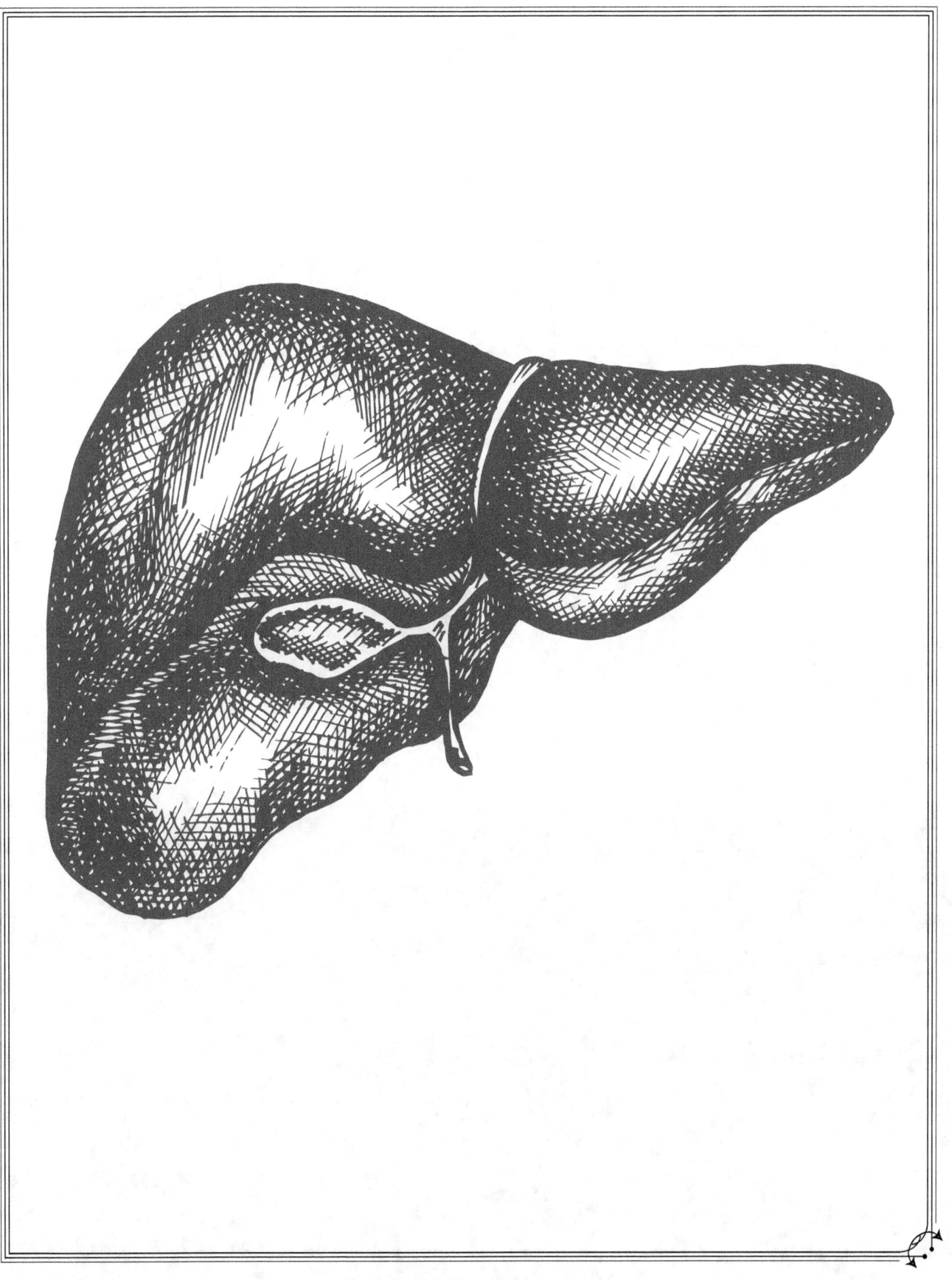

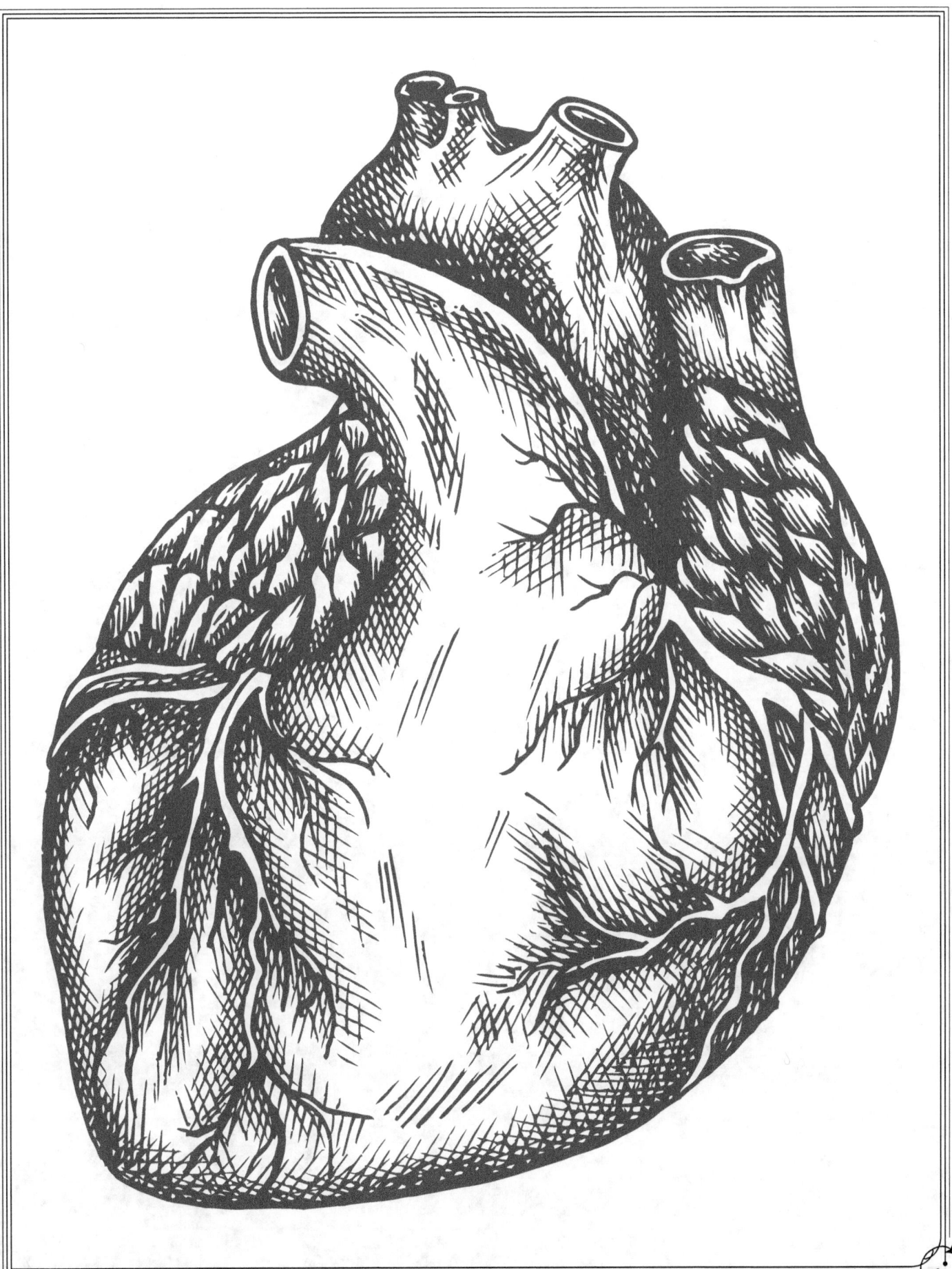

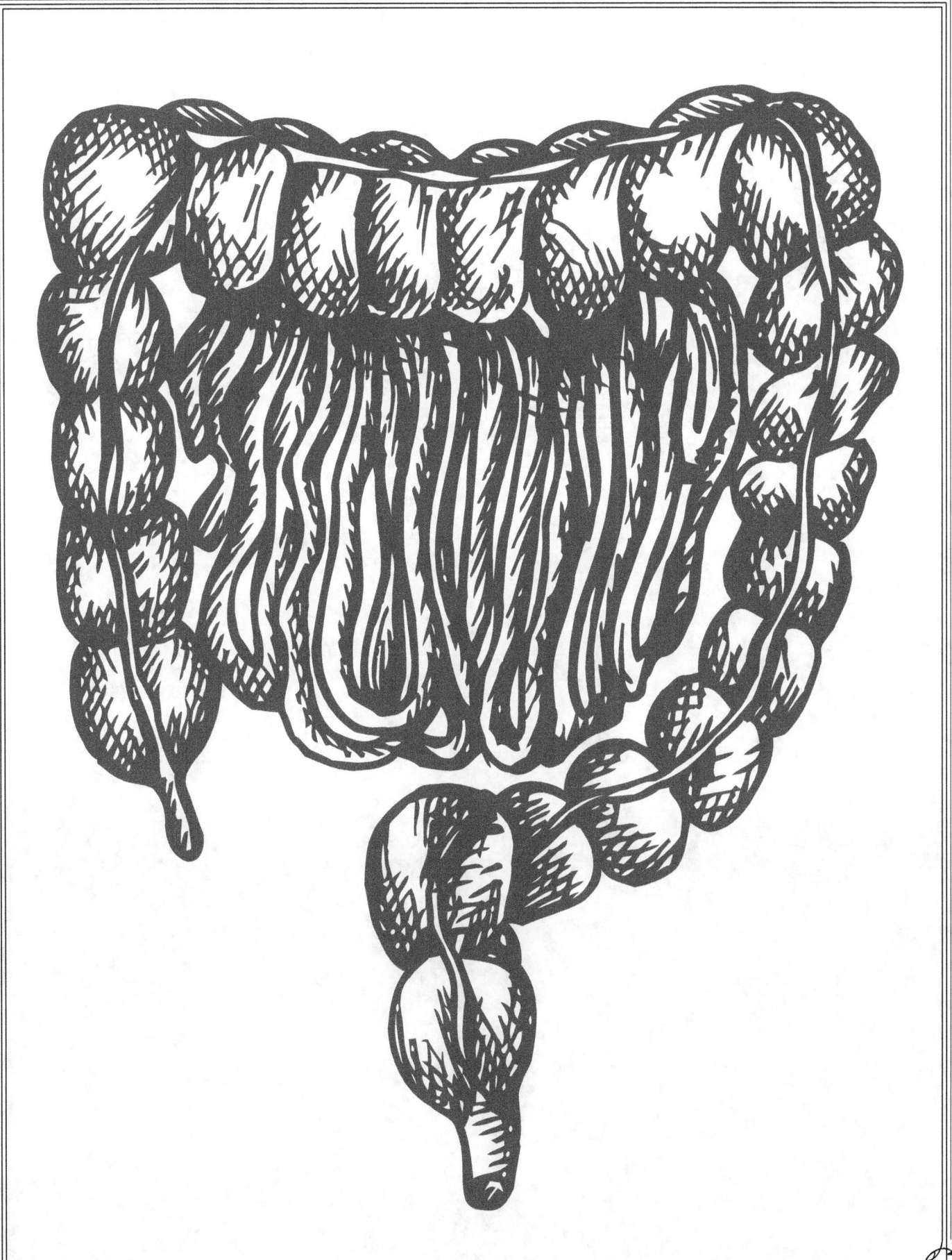

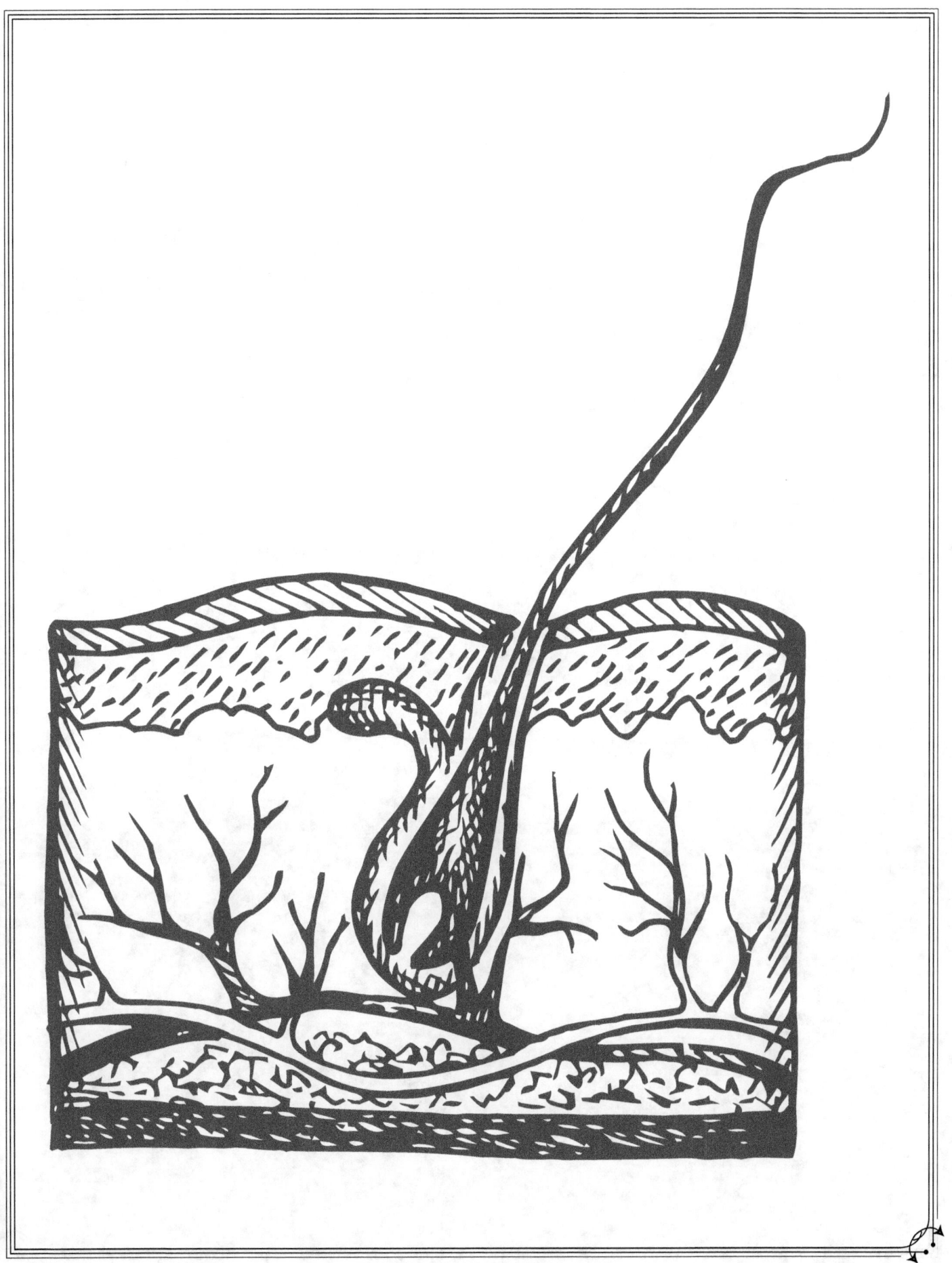

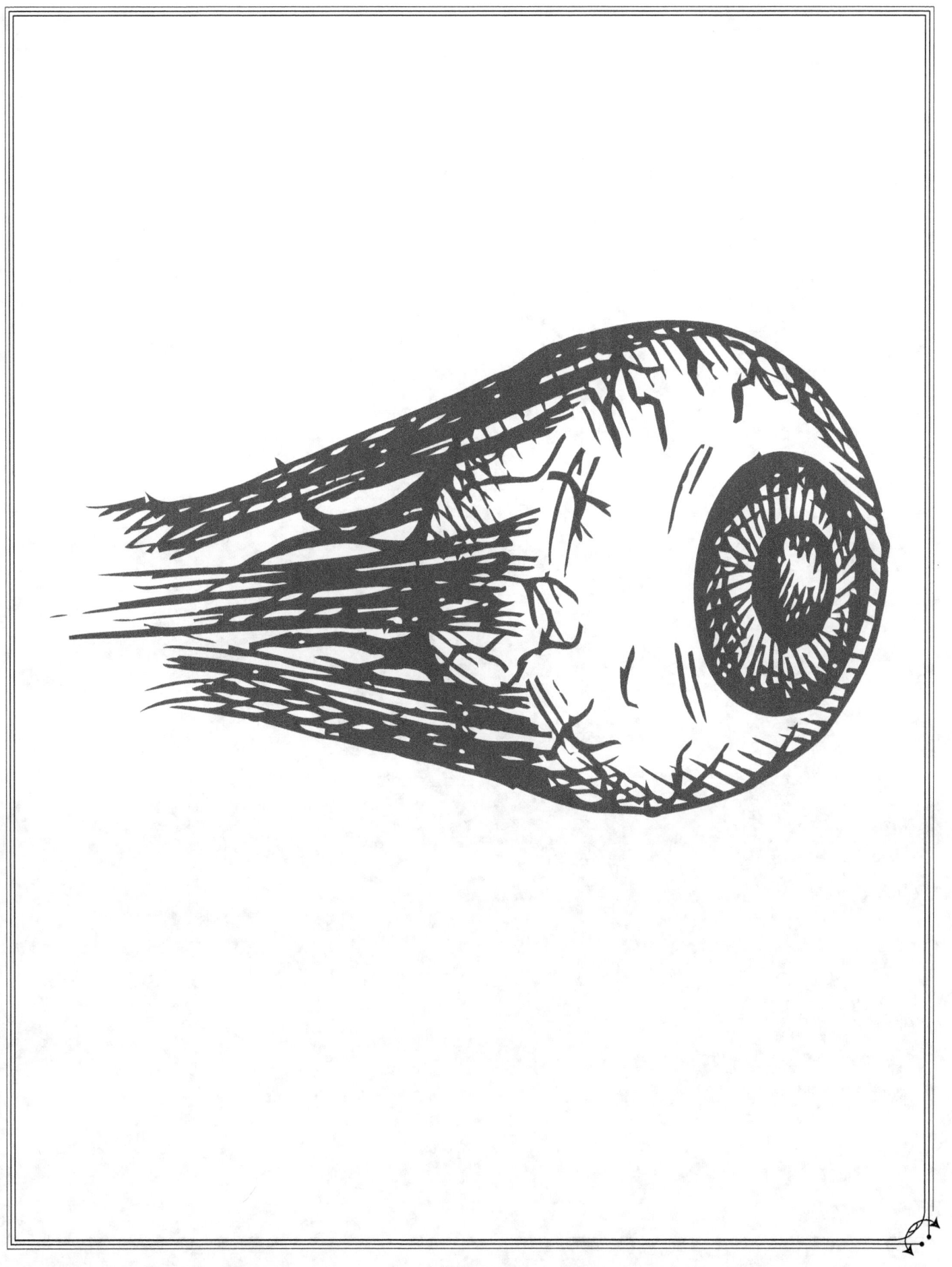

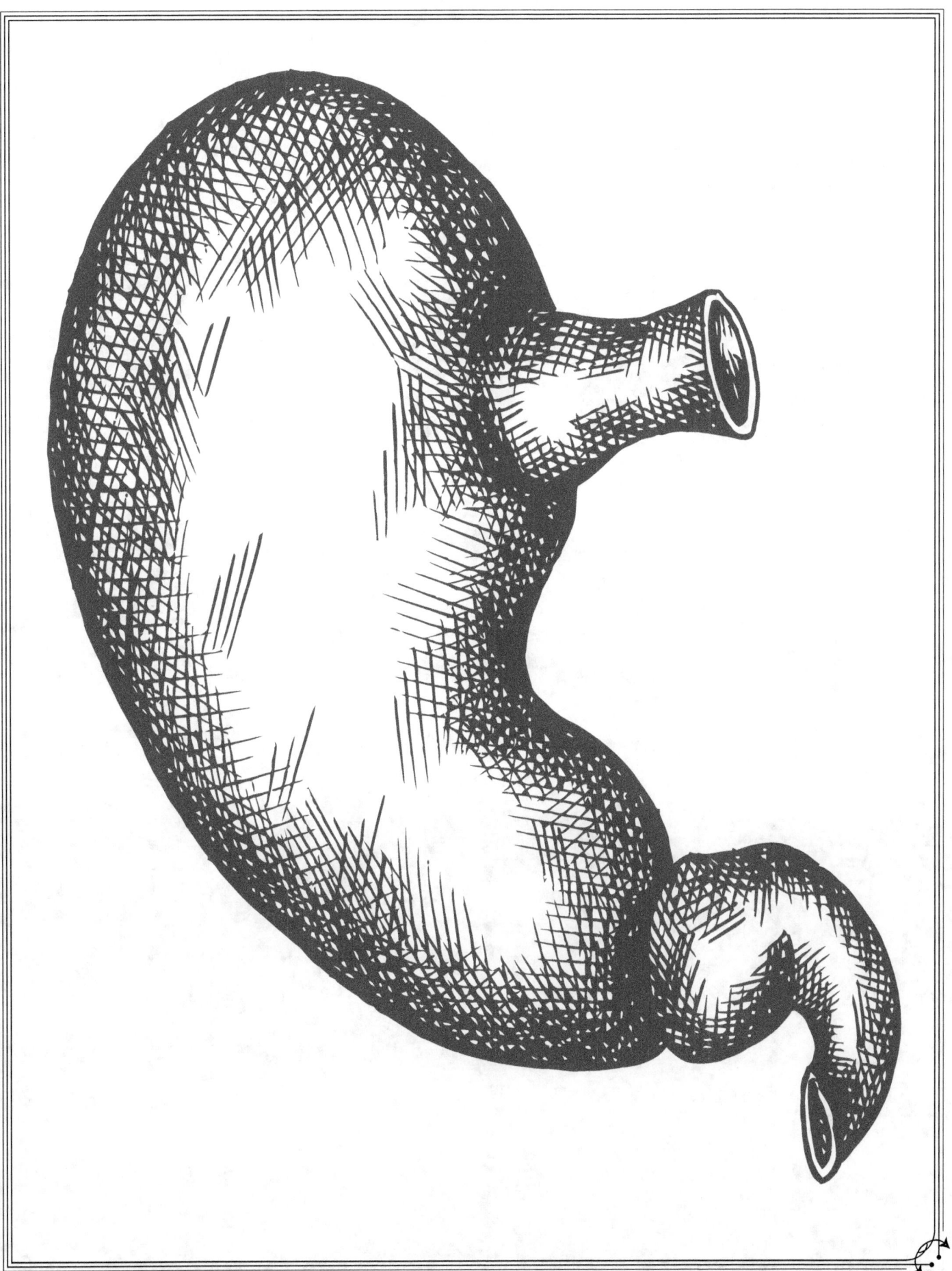

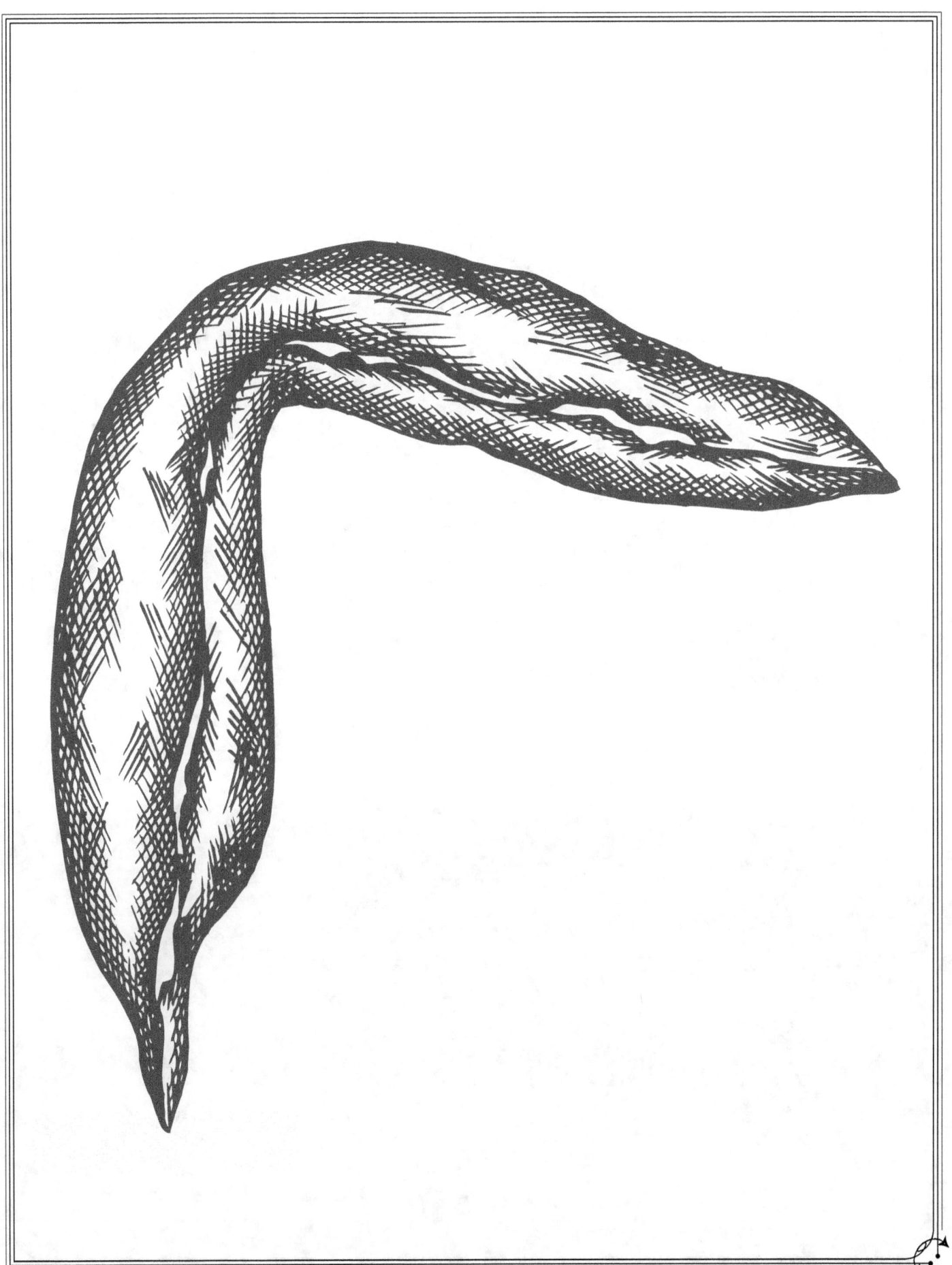

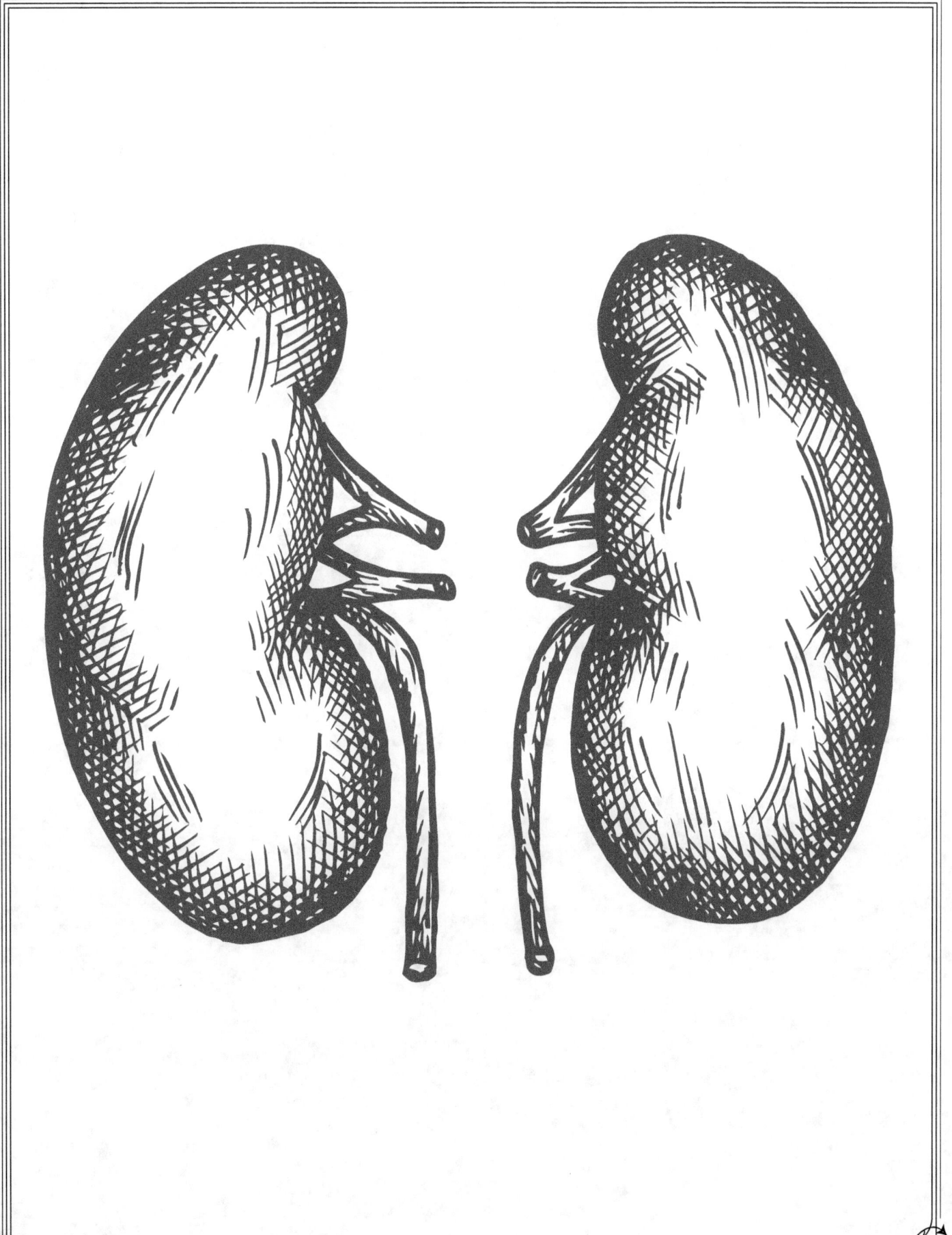

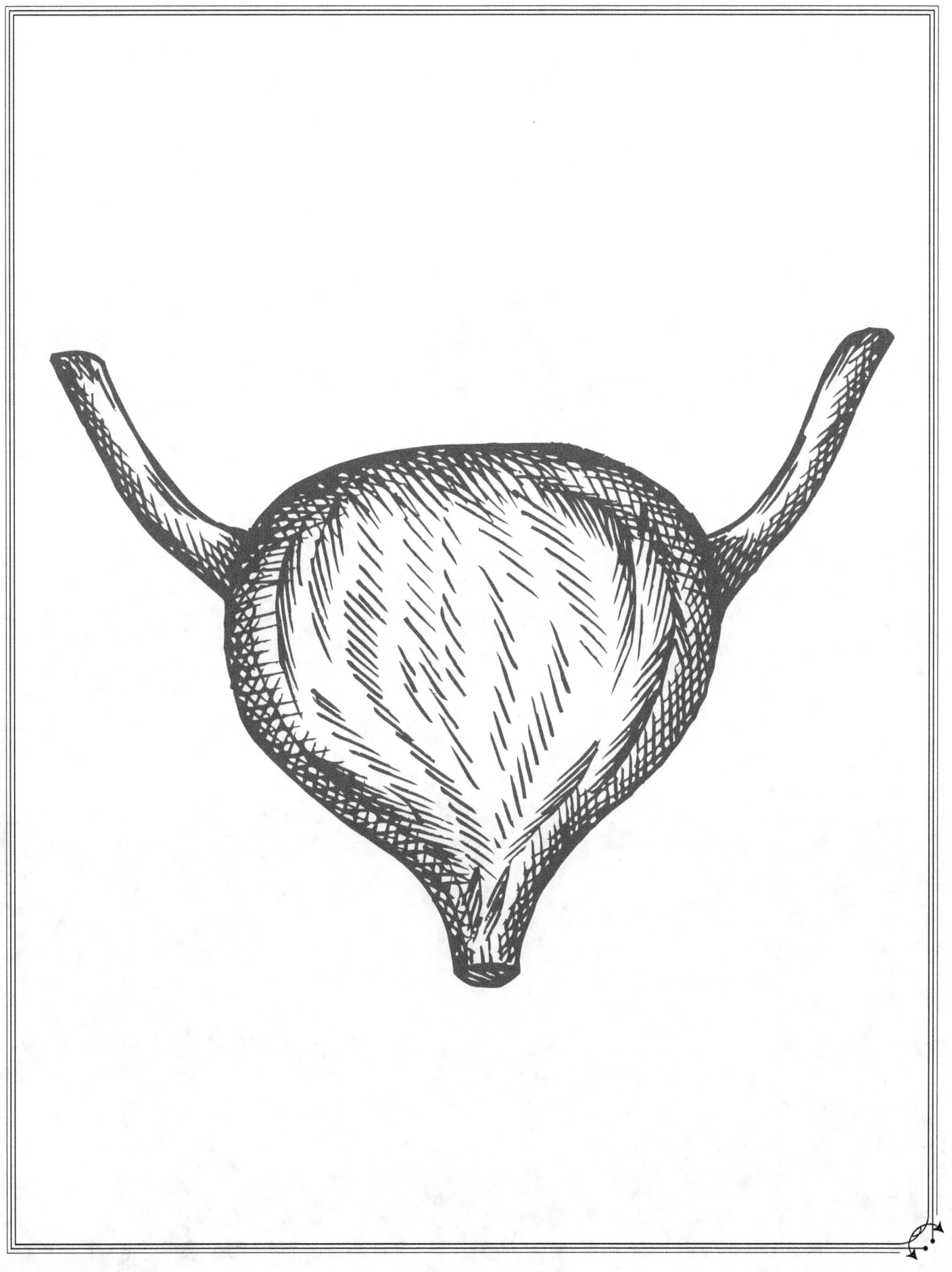

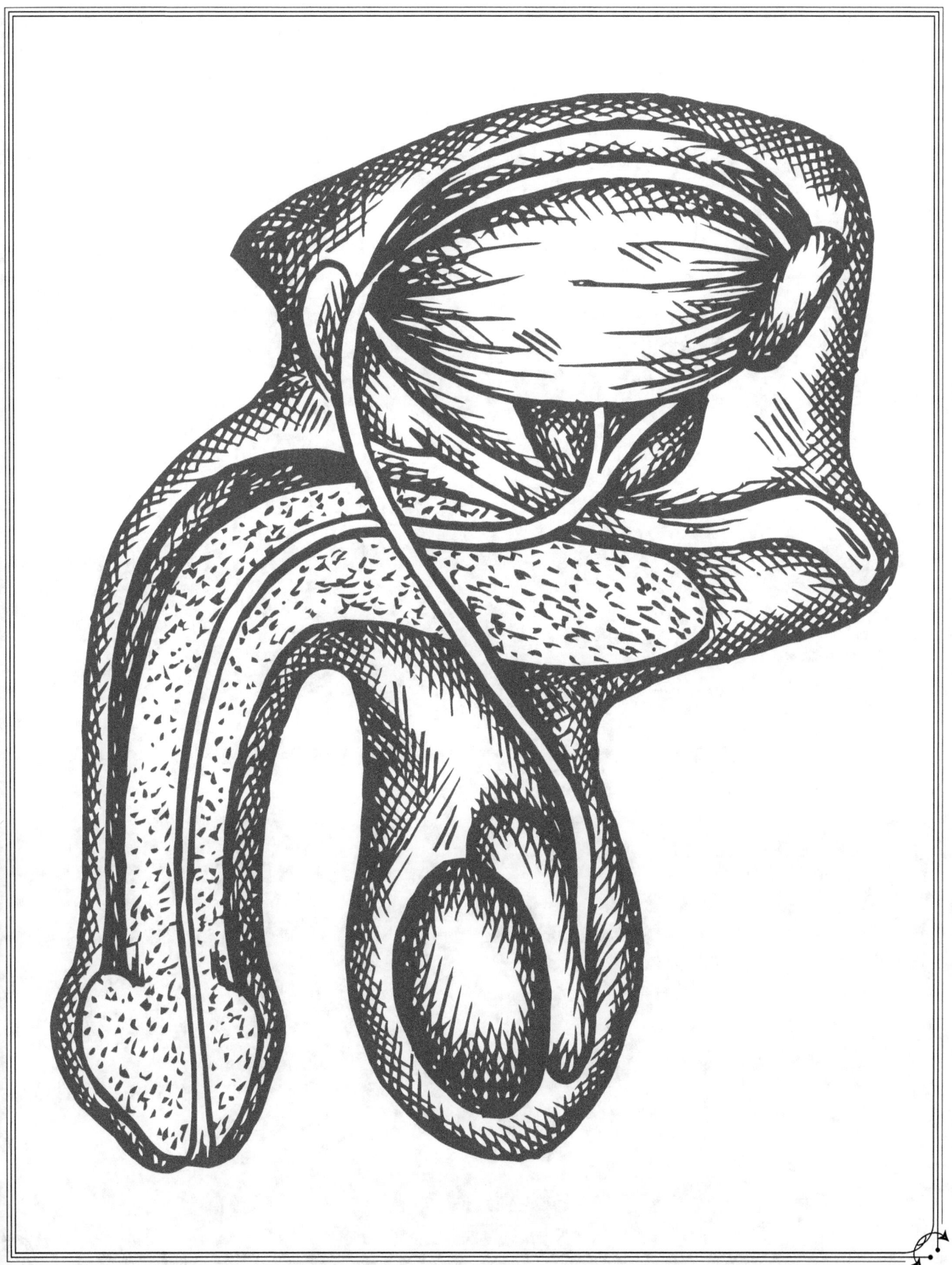

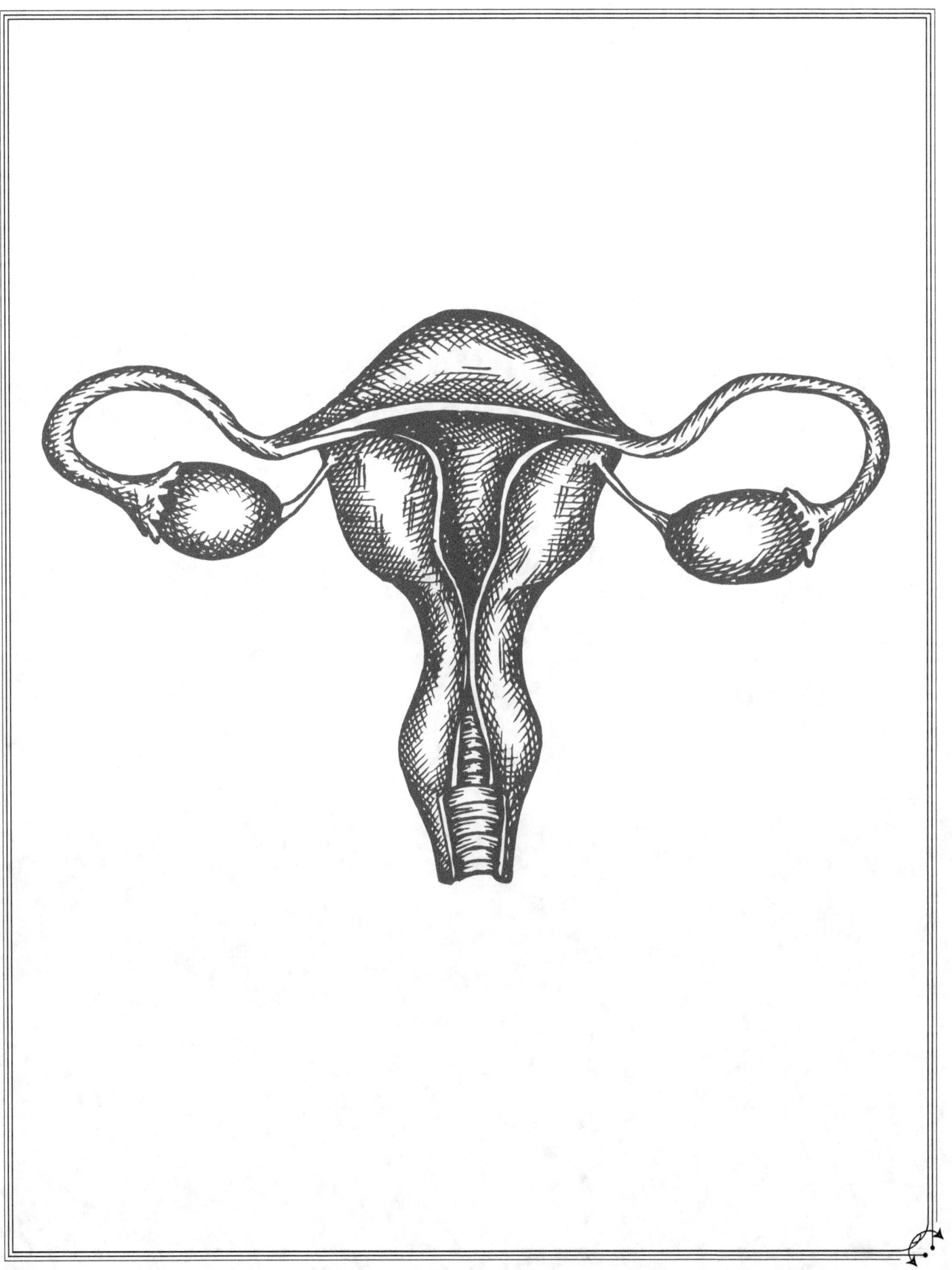

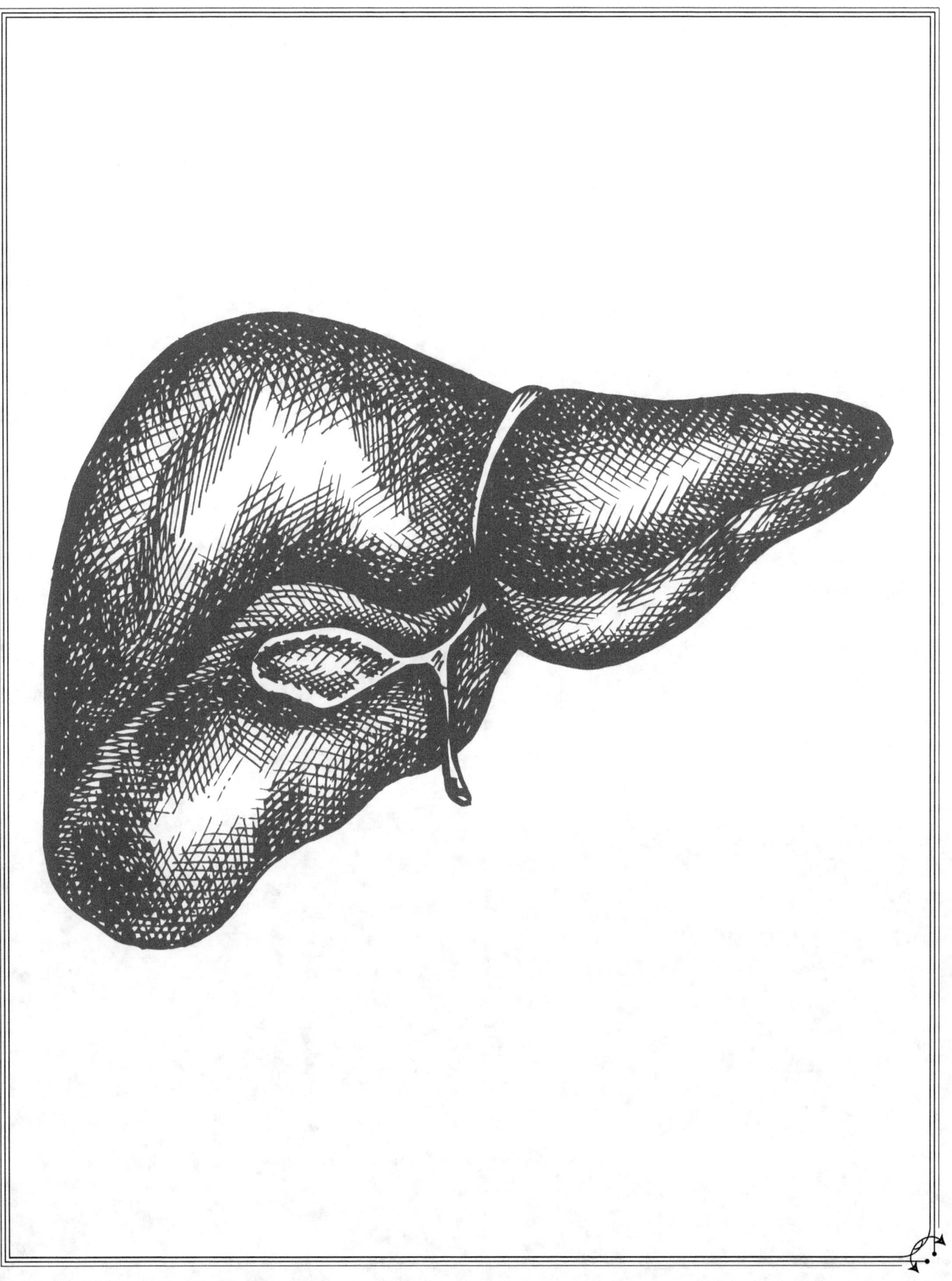

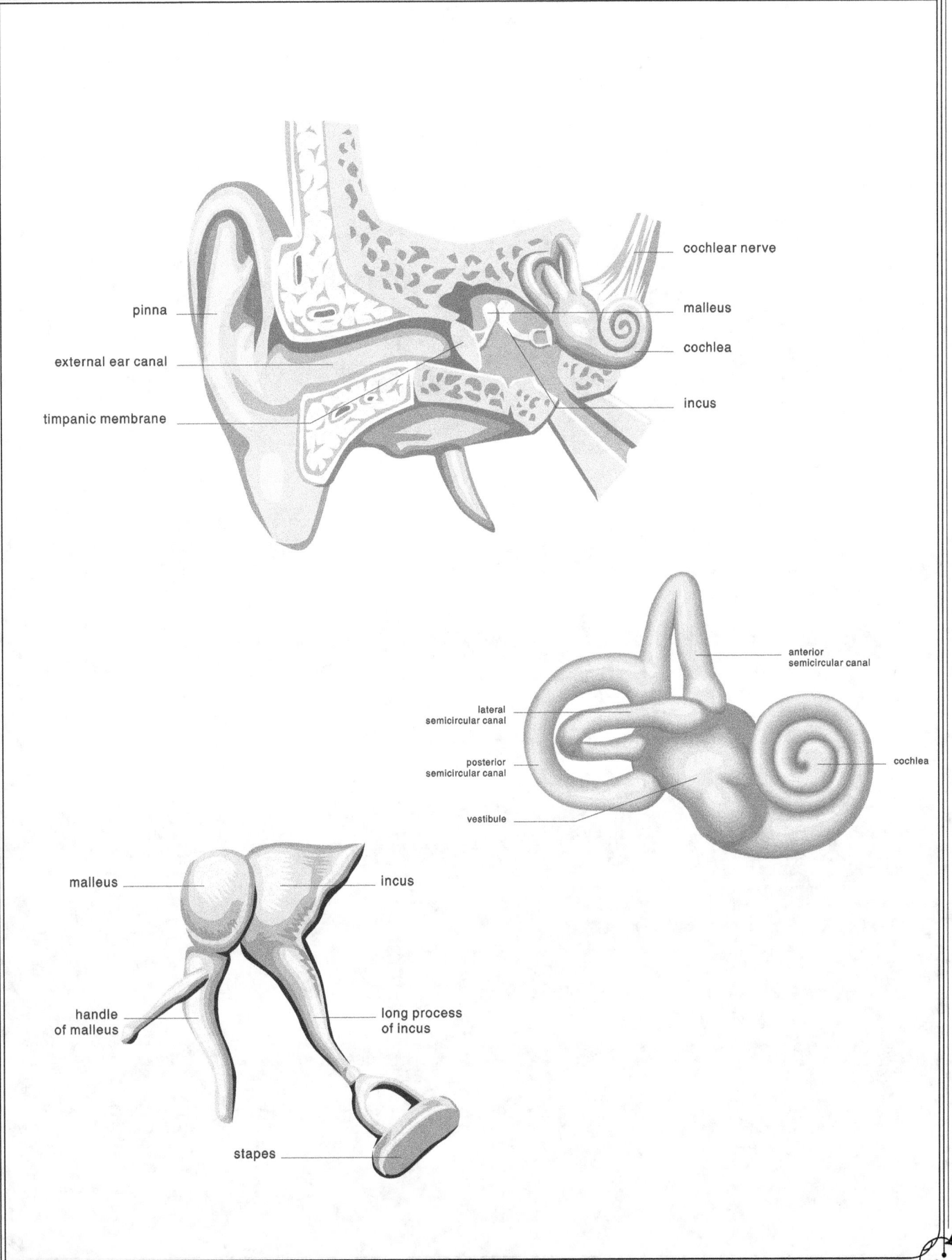

cochlear nerve

pinna

malleus

external ear canal

cochlea

timpanic membrane

incus

anterior
semicircular canal

lateral
semicircular canal

cochlea

posterior
semicircular canal

vestibule

malleus

incus

handle
of malleus

long process
of incus

stapes

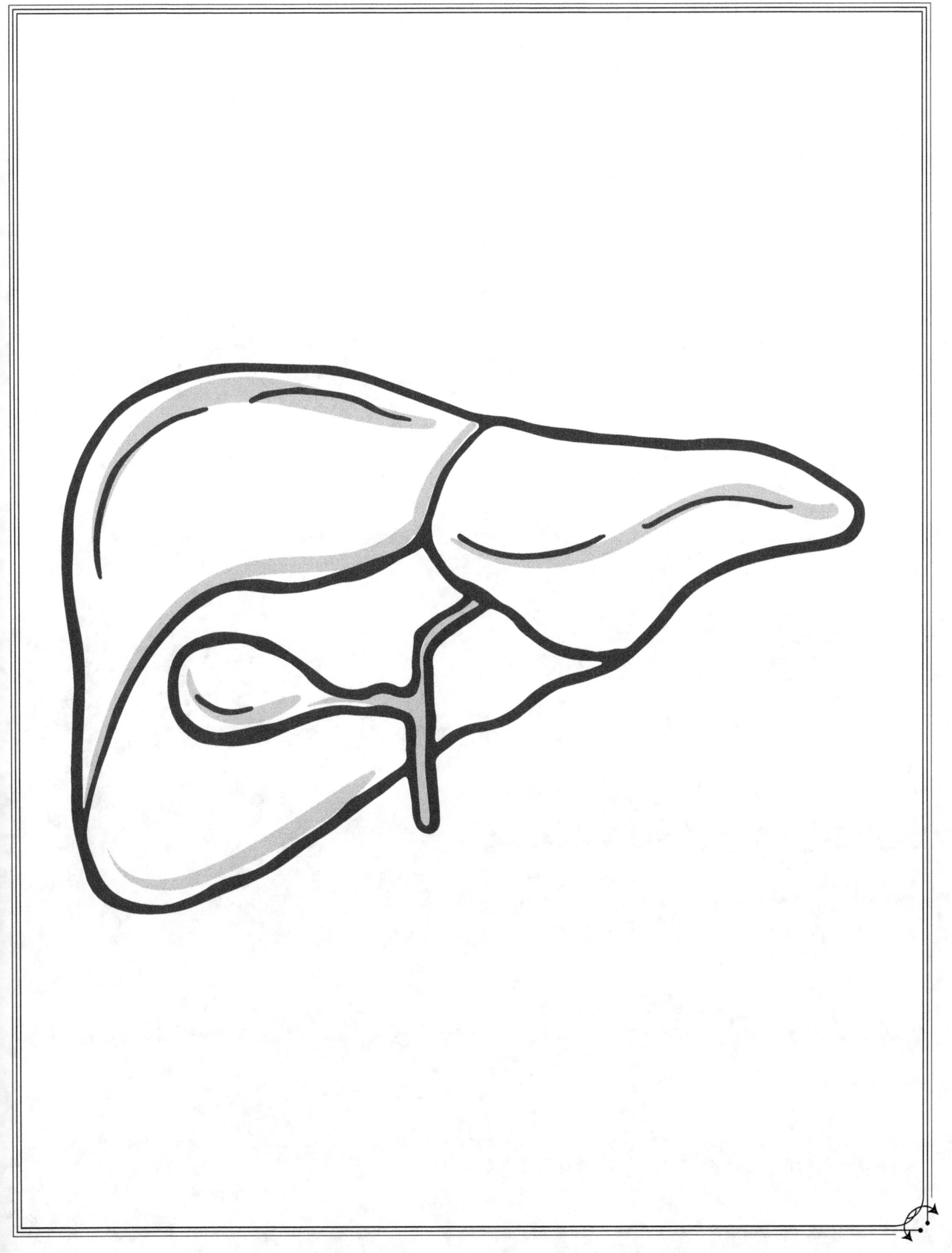

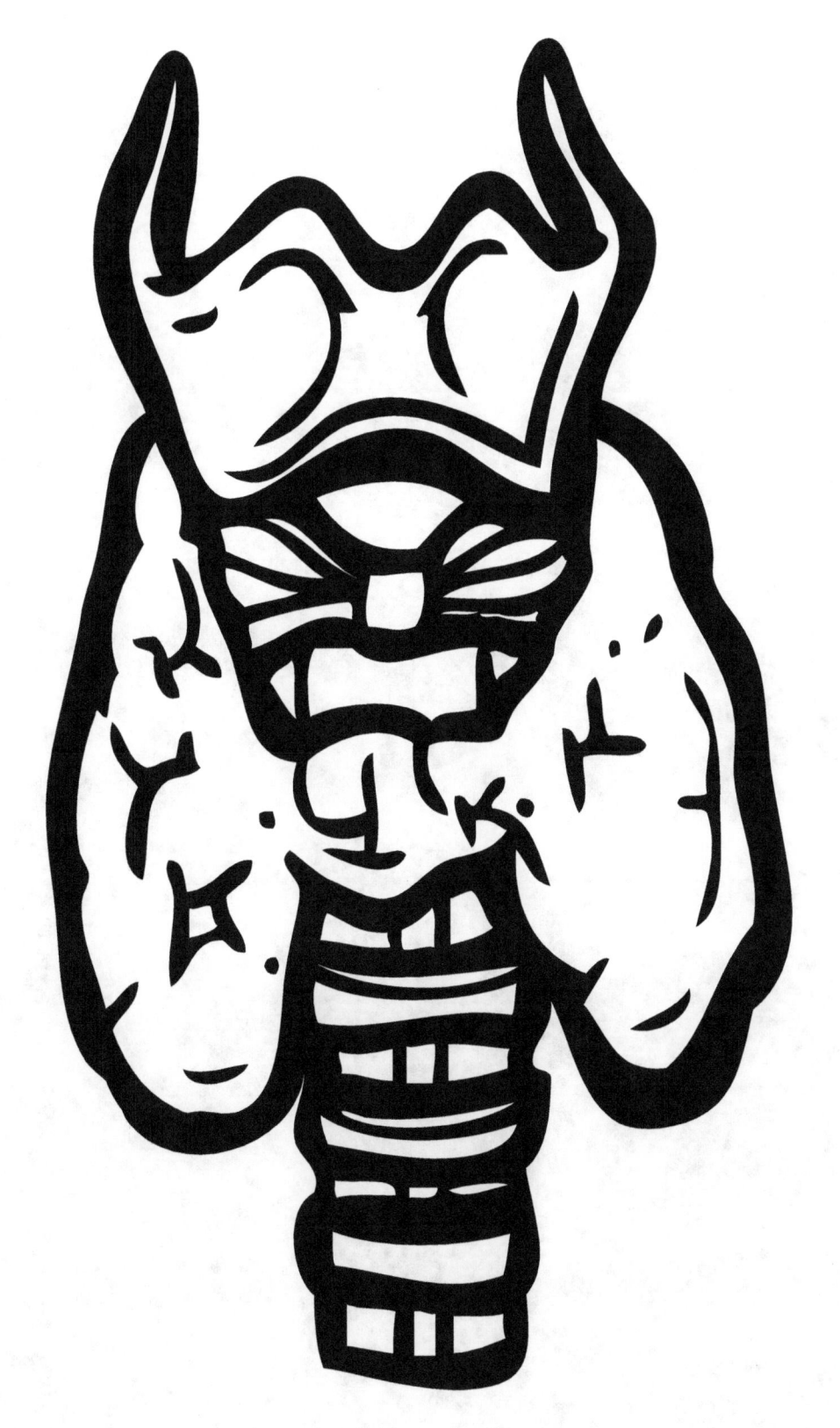

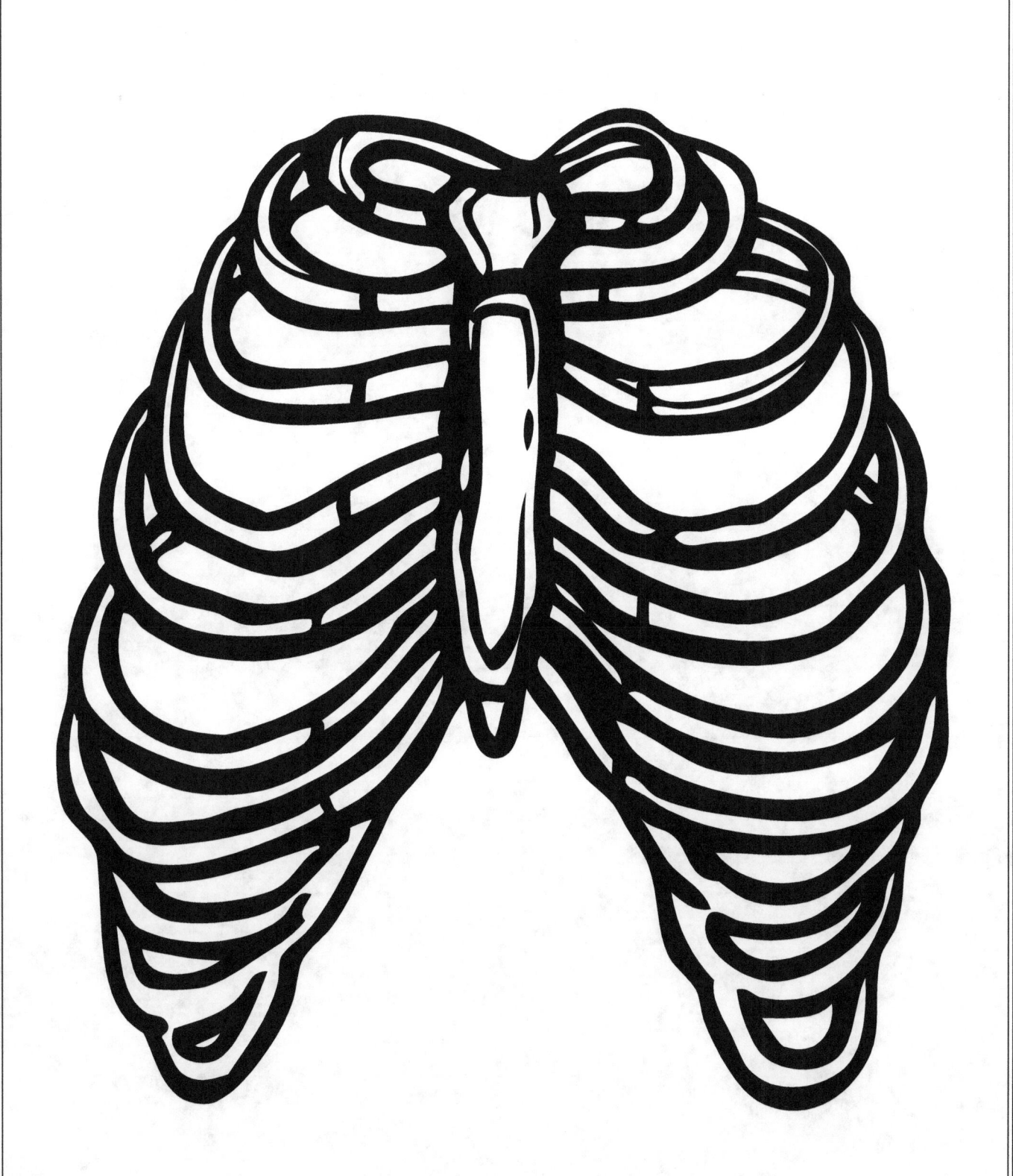

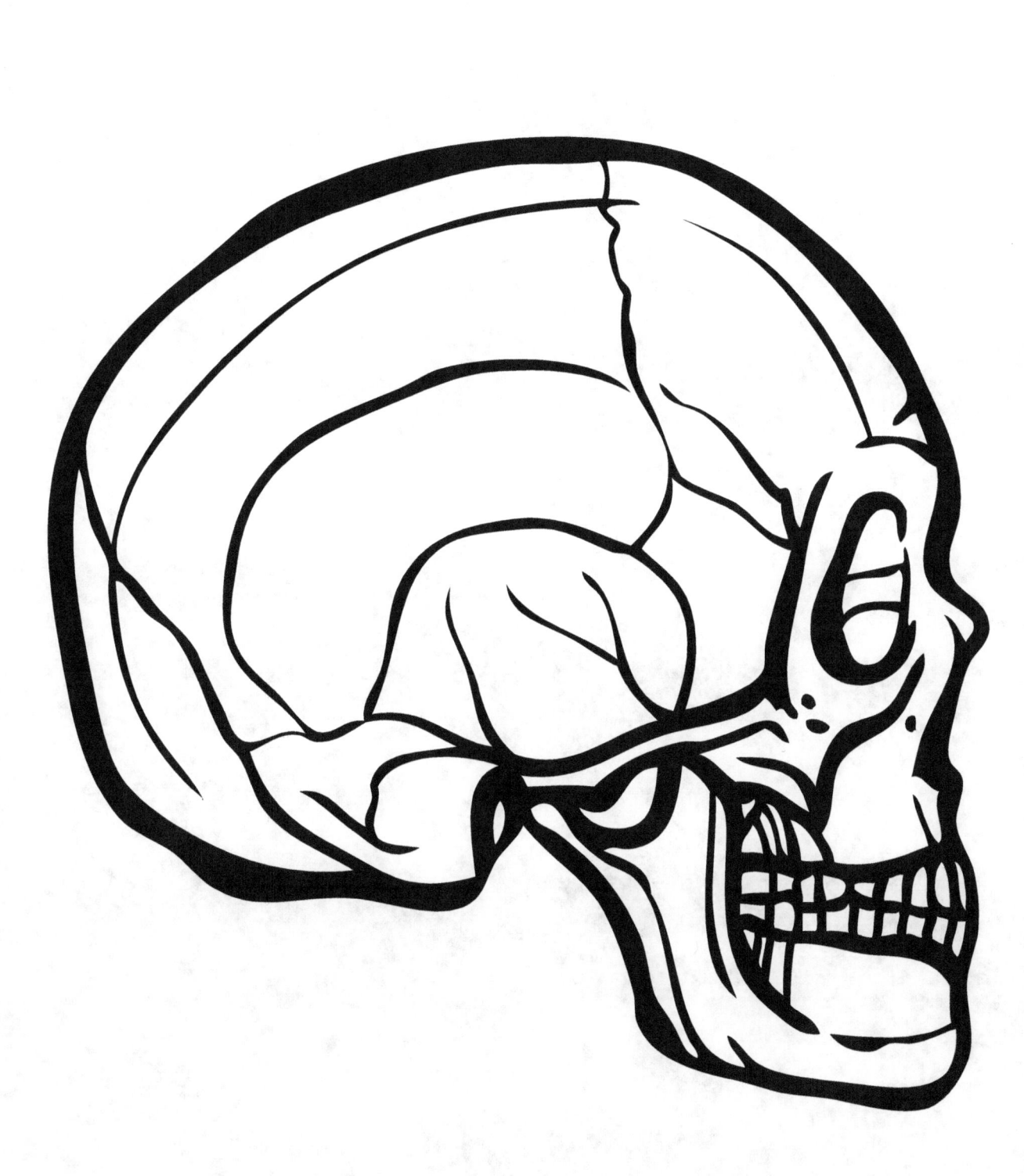

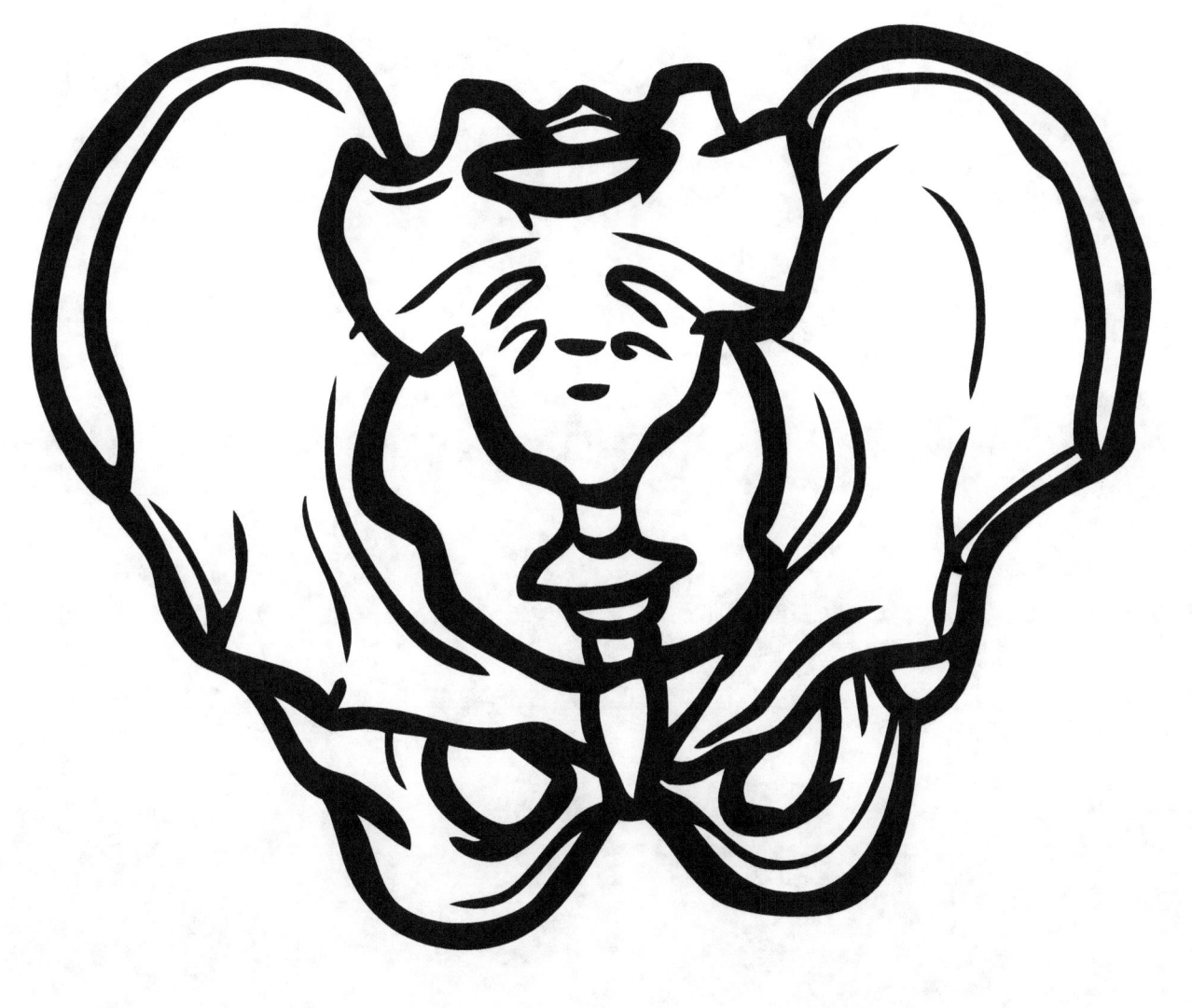

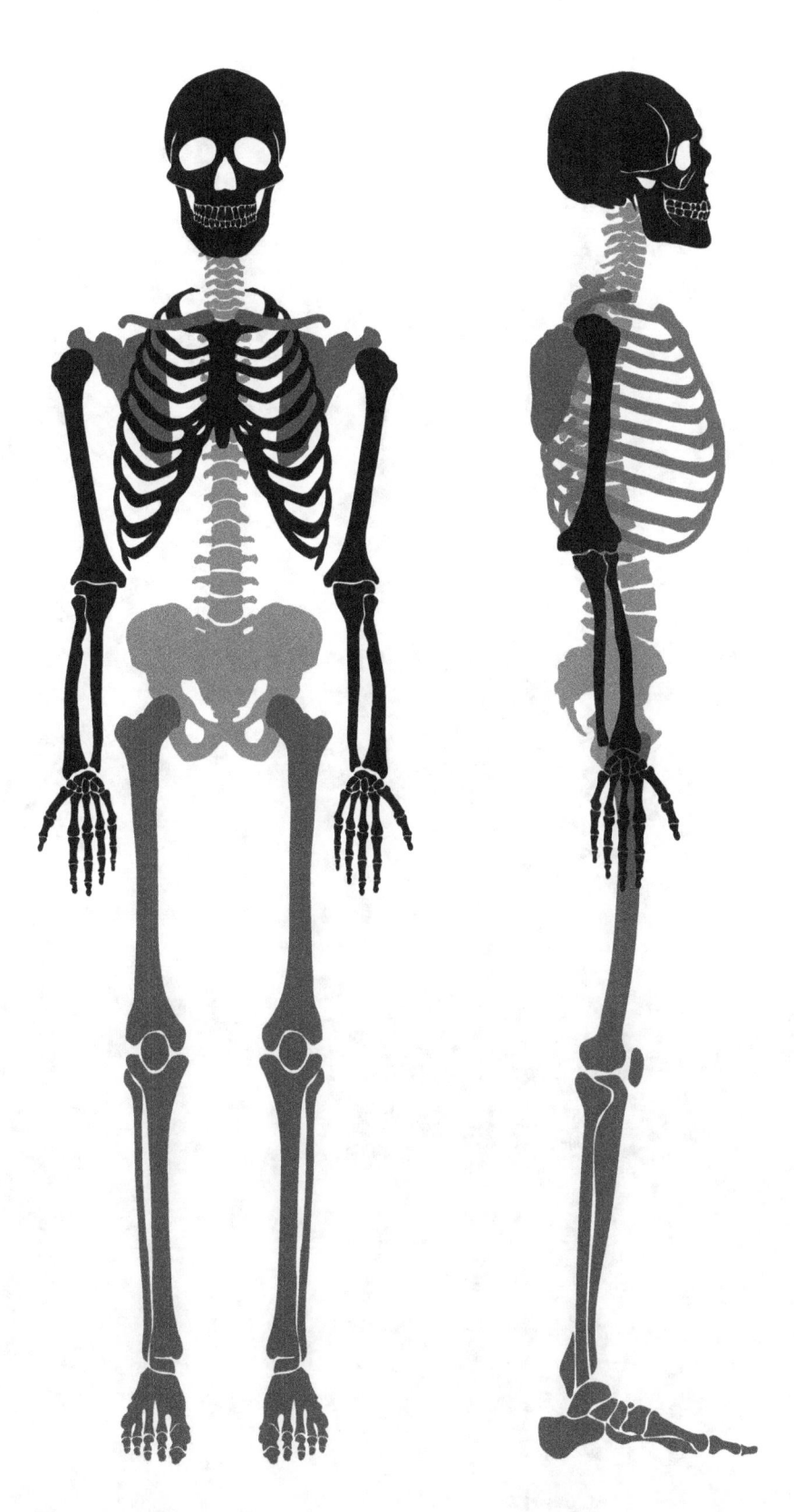

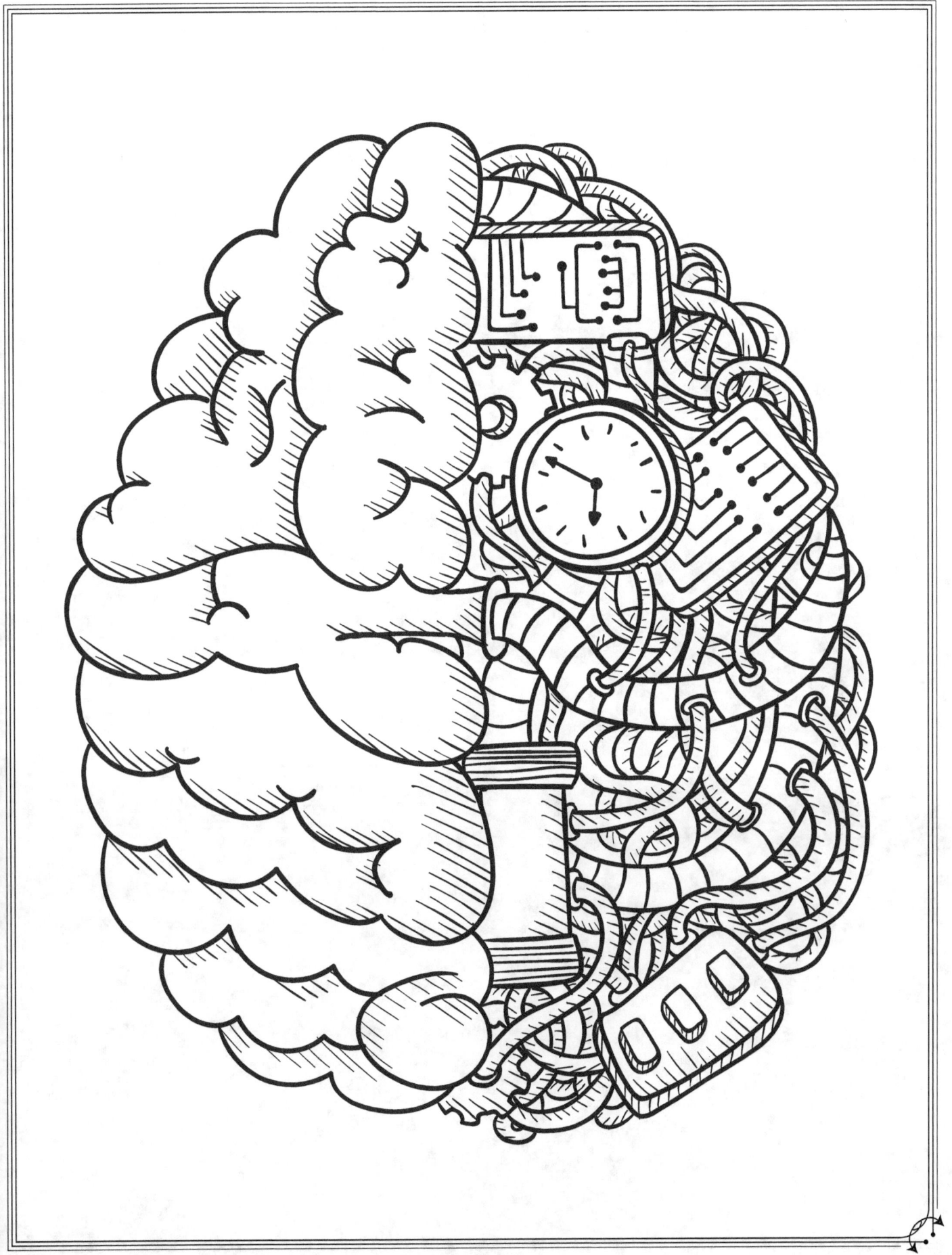

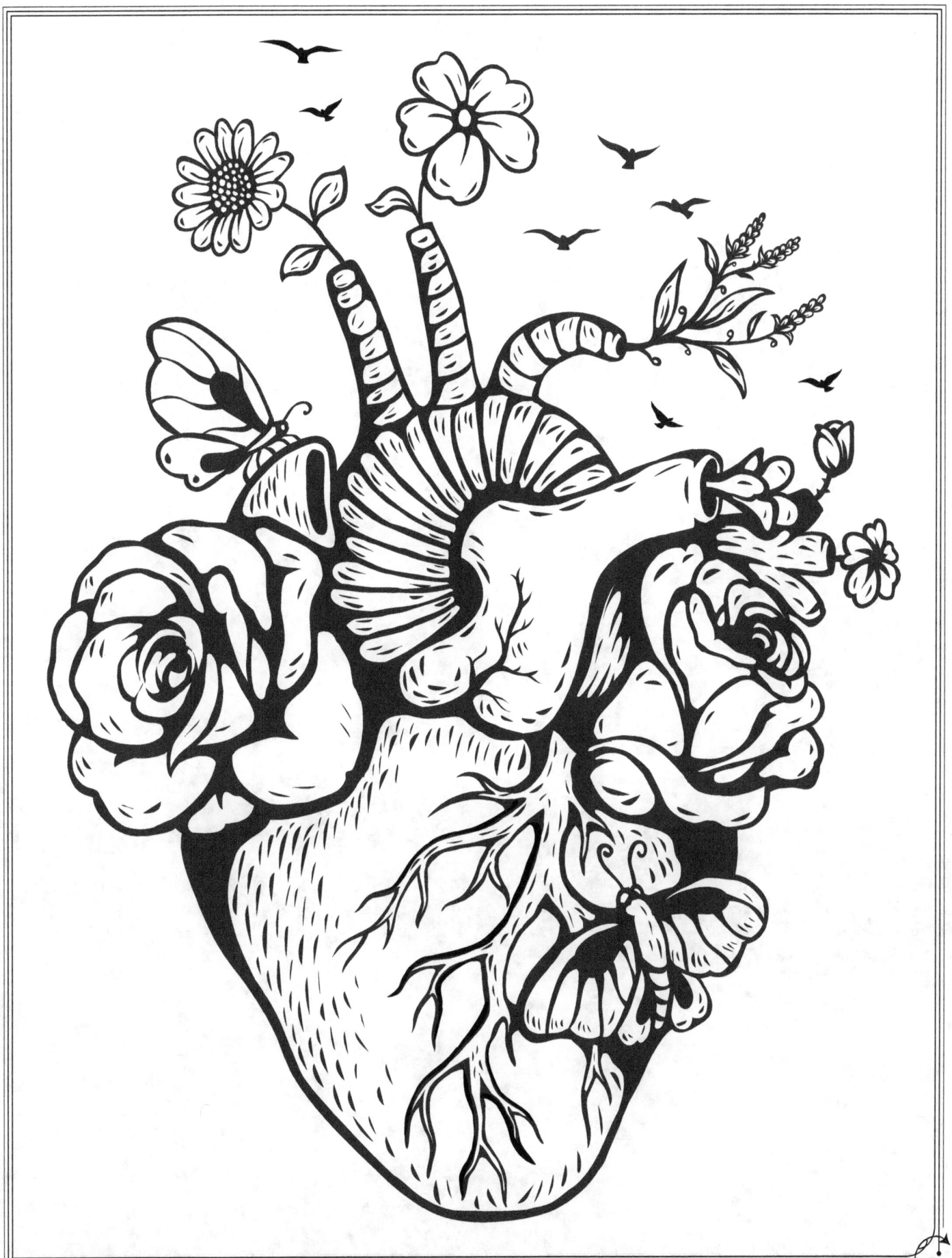

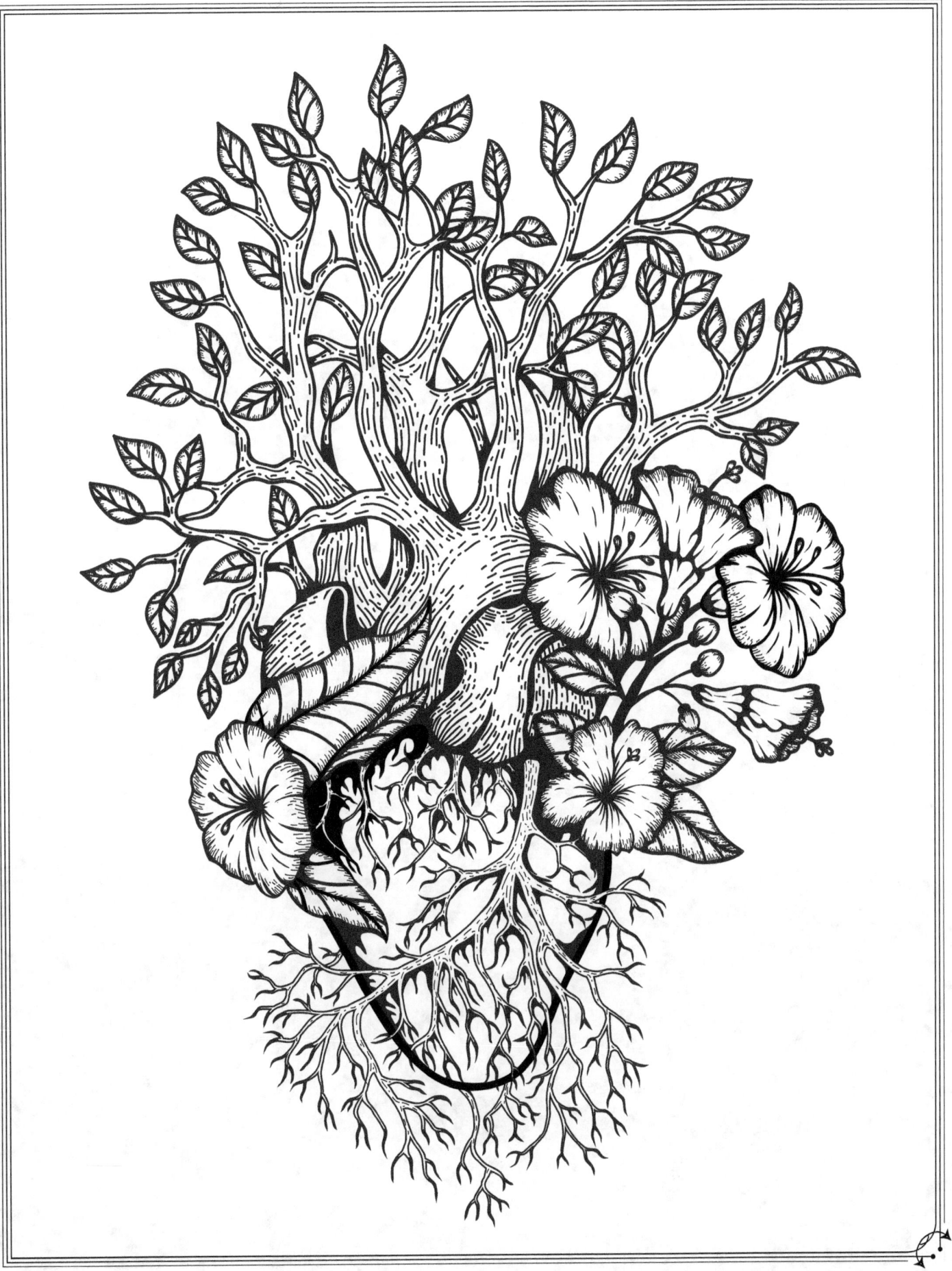